little red book of
mindfulness

little red book of
mindfulness

JOHN OAKLEY MCELHENNEY

Press of Light and Space ● Austin, Texas

Contents

Welcome Home

You are home. Your mind is jumping with anxiety and exhaustion. What do you do?

In this tiny book, I'm going to attempt to shed light on a mindfulness practice that has been many years in the orchestration. I find these ideas quite soothing. I hope you find in this "little" book a few tidbits to help you soothe that monkey mind of yours. Today, I write as part of my meditation. I've learned that writing for me is very cathartic. Later, if I'm able to read my writing to a friend who has attention for me, I begin to feel the healing of the process.

This is a conversation I have with myself. I hope you can cultivate an observer in your own mind. It can help you "label" those pesky moods and intrusive thoughts. At that point the decision is up to you.

1. deal with the situation

2. delegate the next right action

3. let it go

4. get on with what is next (my choice)

So frequently, we get pulled into drama and chaos by our own minds. I am hopeful you can find a few ideas here that calm your own magical LLLM (Large Living Language Model).

What you are thinking is your life. Your present is 100% mood and thought. Here are some tools to help you explore tuning and fine-tuning your life experience. Get more mindful. Find your way to a calmer life and more health and optimism. I am always here in my mind. The conversations I'm having with me contain my entire conscious life. Beware your thoughts. Mind them. Label them. Train them.

When the bad thoughts or anxious ruminations no longer serve you, make a change: mindfully.

Namasté.

November 27, 2024

Interrupting Our Own Storytelling: a 4-Step Path to Mindfulness

We tell ourselves stories all the time. Often we tell our stories to others. Here's how this might look.

"Well, I tried the best I could to be a great co-parent after the divorce, but my ex-wife was too angry and didn't want to include me in any of the parenting decisions, even though that was part of our legal decree..."

Yadda yadda yadda. I'm telling this story to myself or to a friend, it doesn't matter, it's just a story.

STOP.

Interrupting Our Own Storytelling

Stories can be positive or negative or neutral. In the story above I am replaying a story over and over in my mind, trying to solve or resolve the pain or frustration still associated with the memory and trauma I have related to my divorce. Okay. But I don't have to keep telling the story. There's no real reason for me to keep weaving this self-deprecating and self-destructive yarn about my divorce. It doesn't help anything. It will not change the outcome, nor how I feel about my ex-wife. It's called ruminating.

Today, when this happens, and I notice I'm in storytelling mode, I clap my hands (bang!) and say "Stop!" It's sort of like pausing and noticing during meditation that my thoughts have become distracted again. I need to return to the breath, in meditation. In my storytelling exercise, my return is to my own moment of the "now."

"I am telling a story." I say. This is the first step of awareness. Noticing that the story has begun.

The second step is interrupting the oration in my head or externally to another person. Pause the story. "Stop!"

I can then notice what I am feeling. I can check in with my mood. And label that. "At this moment, I'm angry and a bit bored," I can tell myself. Again, I'm labeling the mood, not trying to change it, not passing judgment about my mood.

Finally, I can ask myself, in the moment, "What is the next right action, for me?"

At this point, I have choices. Do I want to continue telling the story? Do I want to stop telling my story and check in with the feelings and mood that is present in my body-mind-spirit? Do I want to go for a walk and change my surroundings? Do I want to do an activity to interrupt the storytelling and move my actual life towards a positive action that leads to a positive outcome?

What Is The Next Right Action?

It is important for us mood-driven people to get clear on this point: no matter how you feel, you have got to get your shit done.

For me, in the past that has involved family commitments,

job commitments, tennis commitments, just basically getting my stuff done. Also me in the past, I could let a blue mood derail my plans for an entire day, an entire weekend, a season. I could fall down the depression hole and get very little done. These were things that involved other people counting on me. My DONE or NOT DONE had a huge impact on my wife, my kids, my manager at work, my tennis partners.

What I've learned over time is this: interrupting a mood is possible. Resetting my day toward ACTION regardless of my feelings. Moving on, taking concrete steps toward what needs to get done. That's the trick.

The practice above involves 4 steps.

1. Noticing
2. Interrupting
3. Labeling
4. Deciding to take the next right action

These are the major steps to recovering a mindful centeredness at any time. I may not WANT to do my job today. I may not feel like playing tennis this evening. I may feel like I need to take the afternoon and evening off... That's a choice. I can STOP the story I'm telling myself.

"I am sad. I am missing my kids. My kids never respond to me when I ask them to lunch or breakfast or dinner. I am angry. I am sad. They don't love me. They don't respect me. I'm not a good dad."

STOP.

This runaway freight train of dark rumination does not serve me or my kids. There is no benefit to "feeling" these feelings and allowing them to wreck my productivity and success at my job. So, I stop the story. I label how I'm feeling in this moment. (hungry, tired, sad) And then I take the next right action.

Making Choices In the Present Moment

Here's what I see are my potential next actions.

- Brew a stiff cup of coffee and dig into the work
- Go for a walk
- Take a nap
- Do something fun
- Call someone I want to connect with
- Write
- Do some mind-mapping around my goals for the coming New Year

- Keep spiraling down my feelings of disappointment at my kids' lack of response from yesterday

- Get mad at my kids for not responding

- Pause, and meditate for 15 minutes to recenter and reset

Do you have a good handle on the activities you can do when you need to stop circular thinking? Can you have a ready list of "next right actions" that are similar, yet slightly different, from your to-do list?

Making a Change, Setting a New Habit

Changing a habit is not easy. It takes focus, commitment, and resetting. I don't always see my ruminations, and I can lose hours in a daydream if I'm not paying attention to the moment and my place in it. I am working on this practice for myself, right now. It's not a habit yet. But I'm becoming more aware of my wandering mind and its powerful storytelling feature, that can derail my serenity.

The power of awareness in this very moment is a key focus point.

- In any situation, I can STOP and check in with my body.

- I can pay attention to my energy levels throughout the day and use micro-corrections to keep myself in positive motion.

Take control of your thoughts and actions by pausing in the moment and recentering then resetting your trajectory. Aim for your long-range goals. Make concrete progress toward your immediate goals. And stay the course.

Defining a Path

Where do you want to go in your life?

If you don't have a good idea of where you want to go, everything else in your life is a bit harder. By understanding your "purpose" (whatever you want that to mean) it can become more clear if an action is toward or away from your goal. It's best to explain this with an example.

I want to be a successful writer. That's one of my overarching goals. So, when I have a weekend ahead of me, I have options. If I blow through my weekend without much writing, I've made decisions and actions that are not aligned with my goal. By understanding this about myself, I try and put "writing" moments in every day. Little steps along the journey of becoming.

In fact, I already am a writer. I write. I have books. I'm writing at this very moment.

Of course, we can't stay "on task" every free moment in our lives. The choices we make have more influences, partners and connecting with them, rest and recovery, exercise, prayer and meditation. It's easy to blow through a weekend or a weeknight without any creative cycles. If this becomes a habit, then my quest to become a "writer" is not being served.

When I'm in flow (writing with joy) I am experiencing a little bit of nirvana here on Earth. Nirvana is inside you. It is 100% in your mind. Unlocking it, feeling it, requires some intention, and then action can flow in alignment with your intention.

First, we've got to define a path for our efforts. Here are a few more of my overriding objectives:

- be a great father to my children.
- be a strong and supportive partner
- walk my daily path with joy and compassion
- enjoy my work
- be intentional with my play
- love life to the fullest

Listening to myself and turning for the journey ahead.

Ambition vs. Contentment: A Creative Dilemma for Life

The scene: I was on tour with a band in Los Angeles and a fan had offered to drive Michael (another musician playing at the International Pop Overthrow Festival) and me to the next venue. During the course of the drive, we were talking about music, creativity, and life. This woman asked a random yet infinitely profound question, "Which is more important to you, ambition or contentment?"

Michael answered easily, "I'll take contentment, hands down."

There was a long pause, as the three of us waited for me to articulate my response. I remember the song playing on the stereo, "Dream All Day" by the Posies. I must've fallen into some sort of distracted reverie as I sat there listening to the song and watching Hollywood flash outside the window.

"I don't know," I said. "I think that's a hard question."

I worked on my answer to that question over the next 35 years. I don't think the woman giving us a lift had prepared a zen koan, but my mind was troubled by my indecision. I realized the next morning, sitting in a marginal Hollywood hotel room, trying to remember the chord changes to my newest song, I was doing my show solo acoustic this year, rather than putting a band together and paying for everyone to fly up from Austin.

I was lonely. My wife and child were back in Texas. And I was out here in LA trying to break into the music business. Or at least, hang on to the illusion that I was already *in* the music business. It's true, I had sold out the pressing of my first album after leaving my previous band. 1000 units. But I wasn't going to show up on any Billboard charts, ever. No one at the festival of old popsters was going to break through except for Adam Levine. His band, Cara's Flowers played on the same stage as my full band, Buzzie, the year before. And we all know where he ended up, famous and plundering young TikTok influencers until his hot wife found out. He was already a freak, with a great voice. He had yet to find a record deal or tattoo obsession.

Ambition is usually what fuels most creative artists. And I have harbored fantasies about joining Sting in his next "band" experiment at the Grammys. From an early age, however, I understood that I needed a way to make money. And in this town, I wasn't going to be in a cover band, so I had to "keep my day job" in advertising.

Contentment, however, is a state of being that is more aligned with Zen and meditation in my experience. Being content might conflict with my ambitions of becoming an opening act for Radiohead on a European tour. It was important for me, in my twenties, to get a job, get married and at least consider having kids. Except I married the wrong (completely wrong) woman on my first attempt. My second marriage provided the first kid and immediate responsibility requiring me to maintain a cash flow that was unlikely to be augmented by my creative output.

So, there I am in LA, I have a small son and a loving wife back in Austin. The question "ambition vs. contentment" was swirling around my head. At that moment, in that hotel room a few blocks from Mann's Chinese Theater, I was struck by a thought that has become more of an answer to the koan than I could've known at the time.

"I don't care about being out here in LA and being famous if I don't have my family with me."

Over the years between then and now, I have lived several lifetimes. Our marriage ended in an unfair divorce about six years later, my son was seven and my daughter was five. I have never had a song in the Billboard charts, but I do have a song on Spotify with over 50,000 streams, bringing in at least $10. It's a Radiohead cover. Oh well.

But here's what I've learned about my own ambition and my own contentment.

I Am Here Now

Having just passed the 60-year-old milestone, I'm still at it. I am ambitious, yes, but more importantly, I'm CONTENT and still creating. I don't really care too much about not joining Sting or Adam on stage. I am happiest while I am still creating. I am creating for my own pleasure. And my feelings of contentment do not come from my massive success or lack of massive success.

My main life elements are in alignment with my hopes and dreams.

- **Health** – a bit overweight, but fit and active
- **Wealth** – working my day job as part of a high-performing international team
- **Spirituality** – I feel connected with my larger purpose
- **Love** – I am seen and adored by a woman I also adore
- **Creativity** – I am creating music, words, and other stuff at the height of my game

In terms of the question, of "ambition vs. contentment" I'm playing it right down the middle. I'm content and still creating. I'd still like to play with Sting, but I'm okay to play with myself, my kids, and my girlfriend. I'm happy to play and work less at it.

Ambition can be a trap. If we lose our happiness because of our lack of fame or attention, we may have lost our purpose.

Refining Your Goals -- the little red book of mindfulness

Let's say you are clicking along on the path toward your self-awareness but you feel like you're losing momentum or energy. Where there is energy, there is joy and focus. Find what excites you in life, and make plans around those activities. When you find you're on a path that doesn't fill you up must make choices.

- Grin and bear it
- Make changes
- Be zen

Grin and bear it – act like things are fine. Sublimate your needs. Make excuses. Try to meditate your way back to happiness. But it's just not working.

Make changes – understanding life is not all about joy and centeredness, take action to change your direction, don't give in, don't settle, don't give up.

Be zen – if all life is suffering, this uncomfortable moment/situation/life will pass.

Resetting your plans and goals is part of continuous adjustment. Always be course-correcting. Always be asking what would work better, what would give you more excitement, and what would make you feel more rested and safe. It is important to ask questions about your goals and habits. Aligning your energy and readjusting your goals as needed is part of the bright path forward.

Aim at your goals. Reset your plans if they don't feed your heart. Constantly refactor and refind the meaning you want to create with your time and energy. Your actions should move you closer to your plan. When you find your energy and effort is being spent on efforts that don't serve you, it's time to reset, refactor, and recommit to your goal.

Listening to myself and fine-tuning for the journey ahead.

Pause

Mindfulness is not hard to understand.

Understanding mindfulness is not mindfulness.

Practicing mindfulness in your daily life is a process, a habit, that once you embrace and understand can make significant improvements in your quality of life and even your health.

My understanding of this essential duality of mind (consciousness) came at an early age in the unexpected form of a tennis book. The Inner Game of Tennis seemed like an ordinary tennis book to me, at 10, but it was really a book about the duality of our minds. Here's how that mindful lesson went.

Self 1: critical, analyzing, trying very hard to hit the proper topspin forehand, racket back, racket low, finish high, watch the ball, etc.

Self 2: knows how to hit a perfect topspin forehand, but we must override self 1 and just feel the shot, feel the ball, see the ball, and where we want it to go.

Meta-Mind Thinking

Most of us are stuck in self 1. We've got to-do lists, and we've got complaints about life, about our work, about our relationships. The past and the future weigh a bit too heavily on our present. So we're frustrated, in a hurry, often late and distracted, even when the activity is something we really want to enjoy. Here's how self 2 comes in.

All of this worry and strife is keeping you from the peace you deserve. Here's one approach to detaching from the "issues" and becoming more present in the moment. When things are feeling overwhelming or out of control, one strategy is to go "meta" or "above" it. I will visualize myself as a ghost floating near the ceiling looking down on myself and the events that are unfolding, the mood that I'm wrestling with, or even the conversation I'm in with a partner where we are disagreeing on some fundamental topic.

Here's how I put the observer process into action:

1. Pause when you notice moodiness or overwhelm
2. Observe the action and feelings (Ghost on the ceiling)
3. Label the mood or idea and detach yourself from the outcome
4. Let go of the offending emotion "just a feeling"
5. Decide what is the "next right action" to take

Let me share an example.

I woke up this morning to a text from one of my kids asking for money. I felt anger. I felt sadness. I felt love and care for my kid. And finally, I settled on frustrated and slightly pissed off.

Pause: Okay, I'm a bit consumed by this anger, let me take a time out

Observe: I miss my kids. I feel resentful when they only contact me for money. I can love my kids and be angry with them simultaneously.

Label the mood: I'm angry.

Let it go: I could stay angry, I could send an angry text, I could steep in my sadness about missing my kids.

Next right action: Respond with a loving message to my kid about discussing the money on the phone, when they are available.

At this point, I can let go of the mood and move on with something else. By taking action, I have put this emotional signal to use. The emotional signals in our life are giving us information. Even a bad dream can provide ideas or information about what's worrying us while we sleep.

Reset Your Mind

This simple process, of observing, labeling, and taking action, can really move you along. Rather than getting stuck in anger or sadness all morning, I was able to observe and label myself in a moment of overwhelm. The transformation happens when you label it. It's not me, it's just a thought I'm having. It's just an emotion and does not necessarily represent the truth, nor does it require a lot of examination. For the most part, emotions, moods, and ideas, go flickering around our minds all the time. When one pops out, give it a little attention.

You will soon learn that your brain is giving you signals and if you process them into action, your brain will be satisfied (at least on that one item) and move on to other thoughts and feelings. And thus, the cycle repeats.

The more efficient you get at processing these blips of emotion or moods, the easier it becomes to live in the space between the incoming brain broadcast: the easier it becomes to remain in the present moment.

Start with labeling. That's all you have to do. "I'm having a moment of fear related to money." Okay, "fear." I can see that I'm really worried about my recent spending on travel. Actually, my cash flow is fine, I've just got a bit more credit card debt than I'm happy with. Action: pay off some credit card debt and make plans for a "staycation" at Spring Break this year.

On I go into the rest of my day.

Energy = Mood

Throughout each day my energy ebbs and flows. I'm gung-ho for a few hours and then I'm exhausted. As I have begun to get more observant of my intake of fluids, food, and supplements, I have been working on my ability to regulate my energy and thus my overall moods. It's hard to be happy and excited about anything when you're about to fall over from exhaustion. Your ENERGY $\neq$ MOOD, but it affects mine.

The first step in understanding your complex energy cycle is to observe your energy and take notes of what helps when you need a boost or a chill pill.

First, observe. When you are noticing your energy lagging or being too excessive, pause and make a note of what's going on. "I am dragging this morning."

Second, assess what your body and mind need. Do I need a break from the work or a second cup of coffee? Would a nap be more beneficial than a stimulant? Can I go for a walk or a short run to reset my regulatory system? What are your options when you're feeling tired?

Third, take action. This morning, for example, I had several meetings ahead of me, a nap would not be feasible, so I opted for a second cup of coffee. I also added a bit of nutrition as well, knowing that sometimes a second cup will get me too jazzed up.

Finally, notice how your adjustment worked over the next few hours. Did you get the lift you wanted? Perhaps a walk would've served me better than more coffee. Did the energetic shift have a positive effect on your output? Did the coffee poop out before you were done? Are there alternatives to caffeine? Maybe some Yerba Mate would have a slightly better result.

Make notes of what you learn. Keep studying and adjusting your energy levels throughout the day. It's like a meditation or energetic check-in I have with myself.

"I'm a bit too up," I notice. "Let's have some food, and maybe a 15-minute nap.)

"I'm dragging on this work today, I think I'll take a long walk over lunch, and come back with a new perspective."

Sometimes, you need a bit of both. A quick nap and a cup of coffee can really reset my altitude and attitude if I know I have a lot of work in the afternoon.

> Becoming mindful is about noticing your
> energy and mood frequently throughout
> the day.

When I'm shifting tasks, moving from an Excel project to a writing project, for example, I will commonly take a moment to check in with my energy. I want what is best for my physical and mental health. I also want to perform my work at a high level. I take advantage of every opportunity to make a positive adjustment to my energetic trajectory.

Before I go to the next right action, let me get a reading on my energy level.

Defining Your Mood Scale -- the little red book of mindfulness

Over time, struggling with depression and flights of fancy, I have developed a scale for rating my energy/mood. 1 at the low end means depression in need of hospitalization or an intervention of some sort. 10 at the high end means about ready to jump off the planet and requiring, again, hospitalization or medical intervention. In my 60 years of life, I have experienced both. I am happy to report, however, that hospitalization (3 times) has not been required since my teens. It is not that I grew out of the risks, but I learned to moderate or tamp down on massive up or down swings in my life.

A few years ago, I drew out a scale that I could use to get a more accurate handle on any current mood. I was looking to define my swings to myself first so that I could then use the same information to explain it to my support team and family members.

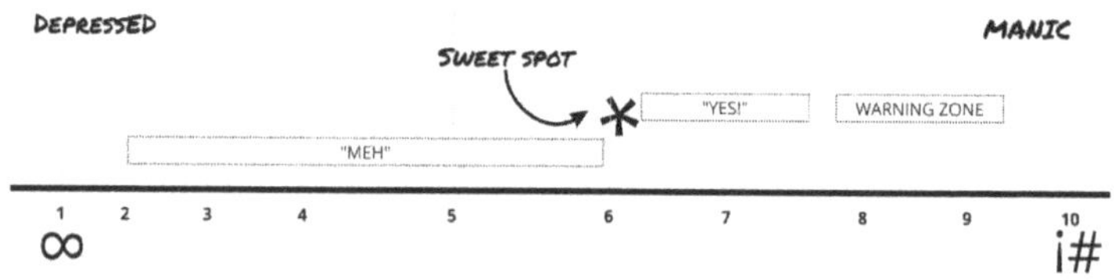

What I have learned over the last few years, in managing my energy and mood, is that what I thought was my most productive creative mode, say an 8.5 to a 9.0 is actually not all that great.

Boredom vs Lack of Motivation

I have been exploring living in and loving myself, in the 6's and 7's. I thought I needed to be higher to be happy. I thought I needed rocket fuel to power my hopes and dreams. And much of my 30s and 40s were spent shooting off towards the moon but never reaching an orbit of stability. What I usually experienced was an Icarus-like moment of bravery and then plummeting back into the ocean of despair.

I believed I needed to be higher to create great things. I believed life was boring when I wasn't on a "creative high." I believed that my creative output was a determining factor in my happiness or self-worth.

I have learned something more fundamental to my own happiness and success: I can be happy and productive at a 6. I'm still a bit worried about spending too much time at a 5 or 4. Those states to me, *feel* like depression. But my idea of depression is unique to my experience. Sometimes "meh" is just bored. I'm not depressed, I'm just not very inspired. Or (get this) I need a rest.

Not even an artist as prolific as Bruce Springsteen can go on forever without a pause. I would experience a quiet period and declare I was depressed. I may have just been refueling my jetpack. I may have been contemplating a new creative direction that had no momentum yet. And, of course, I may have been depressed.

But here's the thing: not all quiet, calm, and restful moments are depression. Not all depression is toxic or bad. Sometimes, depression is just a lack of motivation with a stiff dose of boredom. If I'm tired, bored, and uninspired I might label myself as depressed. I might simply be tired.

New Self-Awareness

I remember a pivotal moment in a conversation with my therapist. My brother had recently died, and my mom and I had spent Christmas without grandkids (my kids) or my sister. In a session, I said, "Well, I've just spent the last three months under a rock. But I feel like I'm emerging from this depression."

"Wait a minute," my therapist said. "I've seen depression. And while you may not have liked it, you did not appear to be depressed to me. You showed up at every appointment, you completed your work assignments, and you even went on a few dates. That's not what a depressed person looks like to me."

I'd say I was at a low point for sure. But she helped me understand how different my scale was from most people who didn't struggle with bipolar depression. "Most people never experience the same highs that you do," she said. "And your 4 might look like someone else's good day. You were not depressed. But, you obviously didn't like where you were."

From that point on, I've been exploring the idea that I don't need to be at an 8.5 to feel happy. The bigger lesson, I don't really want to get "high" most of the time. My "high" is exhausting. It is hard on me and my body. It is hard on the people around me. And it is even harder during the recovery phase that always follows rocket-fueled periods of creativity.

Today is different. I'd say, today, at this moment, typing this, that I am at a 6. I'm fairly neutral. I'm not trending in any direction, up or down. I'm simply being.

My creativity is up to me. My time is somewhat guided by my work, but I have plenty of free time in the near future. What I do with that free time is up to my energy and my motivation. The best part, is I am feeling no pressure to be super-creative, or super-productive. I am content.

Contentment. That's a word I really need to lean into next. What does contentment mean? If I am content will I lose my drive and motivation? Is ambition the opposite of contentment? I'm interested to find out more.

In this moment I am content. I have a work meeting in 30 minutes, and joy in my heart.

Self-Compassion

Learning mindfulness is easy.

Practicing mindfulness in this busy world is the Buddha move.

During the first 40 years of my life, I learned a lot about empathy. I could feel the pain of others. I learned (being raised by two strong women) to listen to and support the women in my life. I am still a bit overwhelmed when a woman in my life is having trouble. My instinct, as a man, is to rush in with a solution. I'm still learning that this is *not* the best empathetic response.

Learning to have empathy for myself has been a journey I've been on for the last 20 years. I did not learn to be good or kind to myself when I was going through a rough period. What my family of origin taught me is that boys support women and they don't cry or express strong emotions. Even my exuberant joy was suppressed.

I am content at this moment. Joy fills my heart.

But, it hasn't been easy for me to give myself a warm and empathetic response to my own struggles. Depression. Weight. Loneliness.

Here are a few of the ways I'm learning to be more mindful in the way I talk to myself.

- I'm fit, but a bit heavier than I'd like to be
- I'm happy now, and I'm learning to be more peaceful when things are hard
- Loneliness is something I learned at an early age, I have learned to comfort myself
- Depression is on a spectrum (mine was severe when I was in high school)
- I roll with the tides, some days are amazing, and some days are a bit harder
- I am a loving father and have always given my two kids 100% of my available attention and energy
- I cannot heal or fix anyone else
- My body is warm, healthy, and active, and good at experiencing both joy and sadness

- A mood is a passing thing, like a cloud, the rain will eventually run out

- Often disagreements and missed communications are better to let go of, scroll on by

- Not everything I think is real, true, or good (but, I'm working on thinking better things)

Having a Conversation with Yourself

For me, learning to hear and modify my inner voice was part of my evolution. Your inner voice is always talking to you, telling you good things, negative things, and random things. The goal is to bring the monkey mind into a more relaxed and calm state and to keep the monkey thoughts where they belong, with the monkey. I don't have to give voice to the monkey's radical and toxic ideas. The monkey thoughts are just noise distracting me from the present moment and the present challenge I'm working on.

Today is an ICE day in our town. Winter has wreaked havoc on Texas again. Mostly, for me and my friends is a few broken trees and some uncomfortable power interruptions. It's just like my inner voice. I can listen to the stress of the incoming news, OR I can admire the resilience of my trees and lean into the warmth of my mind, and the mid-day visit from my girlfriend and her dogs who lost power last night. We're all warm and encouraging here. And my inner voice is quiet. I do need to figure out lunch, however.

Onward into the calm of compassion for myself and my people.

Listening with Intention

A simple way to get out of your own monkey mind of issues is to give your attention to someone else's pain. One of the things I would do when I was feeling isolated and depressed was to volunteer at the local area food bank. It was amazing to spend a morning or afternoon packing boxes of survival food for central Texas families. Often, my coworkers would be families or company groups putting in volunteer time. For me, even if I was feeling low and anti-social, getting up and getting dressed, and showing up for a volunteer session was a great practice.

Another place to practice active listening is AA or Al-Anon meetings, depending on your personal journey. Just being in a group of people who are working on their own issues without judgment of others (at least, that's the goal) always lifted my mood and removed a layer of loneliness. The group circle and serenity prayer at the end was always a highlight for me. When I was super alone it would fill some fraction of my need for touch and conversation.

Empathy, the ability to feel into someone else's pain, is a powerful tonic.

A mindful approach to listening and empathy provides some degree of soothing for yourself. As you can forgive and support others in their struggles, you begin to give yourself a bit more slack and self-understanding. Who in your life could use a dose of empathy? By giving a part of your energy and attention to someone else, you loosen up on your own self-obsession. Get your mind up and out of your own problems. Just listen. Don't advise. Don't tell your own related story. Just be quiet and pay attention to someone else's story.

Part of listening is learning to pause your own inner story. Give your mind a rest and simply open to the words and experience of someone else for a brief moment. It's like taking a break from your monologue.

Ultimately, we are aiming to listen to our own stories with compassion and empathy. We may be struggling, we tell ourselves, but in the same way, we learn to forgive others for their mistakes we can now give ourselves the same grace and lack of shame. Our goal in mindfulness is to relieve suffering by being in love, in the moment, in present-time, in serenity with just how things are.

Forward to listening with more intention.

How Do You Smooth Your Own Feathers

During the course of any day in our lives, we're going to run into people, places, and events that unsettle our inner calm. Here are a few ways I self-soothe by bringing my brain back into alignment with my inner-buddha nature.

- several deep breaths
- walk outside in nature
- listen to calming music (often without lyrics)
- make and blow on a cup of tea
- call a friend
- go to an al-anon meeting
- support someone else's cause

- give comfort to someone in your life

- talk to my kids

- kiss my partner

- pet the dogs

- wrestle with the dogs

- say the serenity prayer like a mantra

At this moment in time, I don't have a cat. (My girlfriend is allergic, so I'm looking for a Burmese.) But, I would put cuddling with or petting a cat as one of the more zen-soothing activities. Of course, you first have to have a cat (have nurtured a cat) that's into zen.

Energetically, when I am upset I am not going to make the best decisions. To the degree that I'm upset, that's the degree to which I will fk stuff up, when I'm triggered.

Recovering Your Calm

First step: awareness of your ruffled feathers | "I'm really pissed about ..."

Second step: is it within my reach? | "I can change this situation by doing ..."

Third step: it is out of my reach | "I will let go of other people's business"

Fourth step: take physical action toward your reset | "I'm heading out back with the dogs for a minute."

Fifth step: serenity now | "And the wisdom to know the difference."

In my life, the serenity prayer has gotten me through most bumps. Here's the mantra I use most often to soothe myself.

> God, grant me the serenity
> To accept the things I cannot change
> The courage to change the things I can
> And the wisdom to know the difference.

Onward into the calm of compassion.

Up and Out

Interrupting sadness and loneliness with a random question or tangent.

There is an amazing global community based on compassionate listening and co-counseling.

Re-evaluation Counseling is a technique for listening in an active and participatory way. I recommend you look for an RC group in your local area. As part of the coaching process (which can tend to sink people into their emotions and release of those emotions) we used something called an "up and out." This idea works even when you are alone. Here's an example.

"What are your four favorite flavors of ice cream?"

What we are asking of our brains is to think about

something completely unrelated to what's upsetting you, and give a list or some ideas. This is a form of distraction. Not all distraction is bad. What we're doing here is interrupting the spiraling thoughts with a task that the mind can accomplish effortlessly. Thus, our minds want to solve the question and complete the challenge.

Coffee Toffee Crunch
Mint Chocolate Chip
Pistachio Almond
Natural Vanilla

And with a simple minor redirect we derail the monkey mind. It helps if the prompt is random. Just reset your thoughts in a different direction.

Here are a few other examples.

What were your first three cars?
What are you going to do right after we're done?
Do you know the brand and size of the tires on your car?

The more nonsensical the better. Give your brain or your friend's brain a simple request to help lift your thoughts out of their loop of distress.

Finding new ways of upping and outing myself.

Full-Stop Reset

When everything feels out of balance, take a pause.

Resetting your goals is a powerful tool. The full-stop is related, but a bit different.

I often get overwhelmed with too many opportunities to do cool stuff. What I mean is, my brain loves to jump to new and *more exciting* projects. Like, I want to start a live band to support my next album. I want to go on a book tour and get a large publisher to pay for it. I want to be on The Late Show with Stephen Colbert, but I'm not famous for anything. Yet. What are my options?

STOP.

In this moment of pause just listen to your desires. Listen to your body. Listen to your feelings of purpose. If you can't hear yourself and your body, you're not going to be able to provide the nourishment and encouragement that is needed. Let's pull apart a few of my big ideas and see how Full-stop is my best choice.

Writer: I've been writing this blog for over 12 years. Why was my Today Show appearance never aired? What am I going to have to do to get Oprah to notice my well-written and heartfelt books? Do I need an agent? Do I need a publicist? Do I need a mentor in the business?

TV Series Creator: I've been building ideas and material for a tv series based on being a good dad even after divorce. What do I need to do to get this one launched? Do I need to invest my own money? Take out a loan? Do a Kickstarter program? How can I leverage my best friend's wife, who's an executive at Sony?

Career: Okay, so I'm doing well in this area at the moment. High-profile job. New term in my job title that gives me more currency in today's market. And the best part, I'm not looking for a job, I have one. But, when is my work going to bust me loose from the grind? Even my great job is a job. I want to make movies, write books, speak on international stages and have someone else pay for it.

Okay, that's enough. And these are parts of my creative life that drive me on. I am hoisted from the bed each morning around 6 am not because I have *work* to do. Not because I have to hustle to get to a menial job. I do like coffee, yes, but the real reason I get out of bed is: I am excited for my life and the future joy that this day (today) will bring. Sure, I'm also hoping to woo the gods of fame and fortune to take notice. But that is not my goal, nor my condition of satisfaction.

STOP.

When I take a full-stop break from all of this striving, I find that I am HAPPY RIGHT NOW. I don't need more money. I don't need a healthier relationship. I don't need to be a famous writer or tv series creator. If I stop and count my blessings along with my breaths, I can feel the joy in the simple being of myself in my life at this moment. I am connected. I am loved. I am happy. What more success do I need to make me happy? ZERO.

If you're happy with what you are doing and you wake up on Monday morning with optimism rather than dread, you are doing it right. If fame is elusive and frustrating, reset your goals. You're already happy, let the *fame* and *fortune* parts take come as they will. Don't wait for the accomplishment to feel accomplished. I remember pitching my first book "The Positive Divorce." The agents and book publishers wanted to know what other books I'd written. Did I have a platform? What was my marketing plan for the book? Oh, and *divorce* doesn't sell these days.

Don't listen to the overwhelming parts of your life. Keep your eyes focused on your big goals and make sure your efforts during the course of a given week, move that marker a bit further forward. Live your life. Write your books. Sing your songs. And if the market comes to reward you with fame and fortune, great. But, if you are happy living your life, the success will not matter.

Your success is already happening inside you. **Smile. Love. Proceed.**

Listening to myself while breathing an easy mantra.

Peace.

Home.

Love.

Now.

MNDFL + MFKR

MNDFL – mindful: actions and words match your philosophy and spiritual direction.

MFKR – motherf*cker: the fierce and direct confrontation of ideas, actions, and words that don't match our values.

It is easy to be a MFKR. It's easy to hate on stuff you don't like or (probably) don't understand. I have spent a lot of time in the last five years taming my MFKR attitude. On Facebook, for example, it might be hard to ignore political posts, or ads that claim oral ketamine can replace therapy. But here's where I've landed on this anger inside myself.

You do not have to respond to social media or the news. You don't have to educate or correct the other haters in the world. It is fine to ignore the stuff you don't like. In the not-too-distant past it would've been easy for me to pick a fight with a foolish post (usually from a high school "friend") on Facebook. Today, I simply block them. No need to have a conversation of any kind with them. Done. Move on.

Walking In Peace

In a mindful approach to the walk of life and social media, it can be a bit more difficult to define and then align with your life goals. I know that sounds woo-woo, but it's actually quite practical.

If you do not know where you want to go, how can you determine if an action is TOWARD or AWAY from your ultimate goal? If you don't know your purpose in life, how will you determine your course of action, today, this weekend, or this year? The point is, you can't know where to go if you don't know where you are aiming.

If you are not aware of your uber-goal it is highly likely that you are not crafting an intentional life. That's what we want: to live an intentional and directed life.

You must identify your goals so you can make strides toward your best life.

But Why MFKR?

You may be thinking if you're following along, that MFKR has no place in a life of peace or holistic health. Let's pull that idea apart for a second. Let's say you're sitting beside a calm mountain lake. You are in a mindful repose. Perhaps you are writing about how blissful and serene your life is. Breathing is slow and easy. As you follow in-breath number 34 an enormous diesel pickup truck pulls into the parking lot behind you.

Three dogs, two kids, and six adults with a Yeti cooler and a thumping boombox unload and set up for their afternoon party.

Now what?

In this moment, as blissful as you might have been, you've got issues. You've also got an infinite number of options.

A mindful non-MFKR person might simply leave and find solace somewhere else. A MFKR would ignite and confront the new arrivals. **A MNDFL MFKR** will explore a number of options in their mind before taking action.

Let's up that ante a bit. Let's say you are driving along a snowy mountain pass when a bigass truck jams up behind you and seems to be pressing you to either go faster or go off the road. Now, what do you do?

A MNDFL MFKR tries the path of peace until his peace or safety is threatened. Then, watch out. Time to unleash the MFKR. You still have a ton of options as long as you maintain your self-awareness and calm. You take clear and decisive action to eliminate the risk to you and your family.

Walking your path, try and be mindful. When you're contradicted or upset by the words or actions of others, continue to assess your options. Then, like a ninja, when it's time to take action, move without hesitation to neutralize the threat.

Then breathe and let it go. Recenter. Refind your peace.

The stickers I made a year ago have started a number of interesting conversations. It seems there are two responses to MNDFL MFKR.

1. Frustration or anger

2. Laughter and joining

In that way, these hearts are like an acid test. Are you IN or are you OUT?

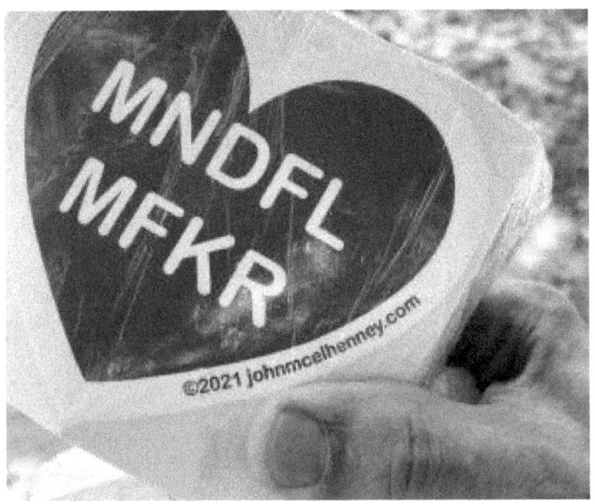

MNDFL
MFKR
©2021 johnmcelhenney.com

Hello & Goodbye

We've reached another beginning.

Take these ideas, words, musings as a gift. Or a joke, if you like. Whatever allows the ideas of mindfulness to float around in your cloud-brain. Life is about connecting, reconnection, and forgetting all we've learned.

Until we return to patience, learning again what we thought we knew, I am awaiting your arrival here.

Continuously arriving at patience.

More Thoughts

Please seek out more of my writing on Amazon if you like, or

on MCELHENNEY.NET where you will find my ongoing writing catalog.

Top Five Books from Others

- The Seven Story Mountain – Thomas Merton
- The Dark Night of the Soul – Thomas Moore
- Siddhartha – Herman Hesse
- Dharma Bums – Jack Kerouac
- The Complete Journals – Anaïs Nin